HEALTHY FOR LIFE

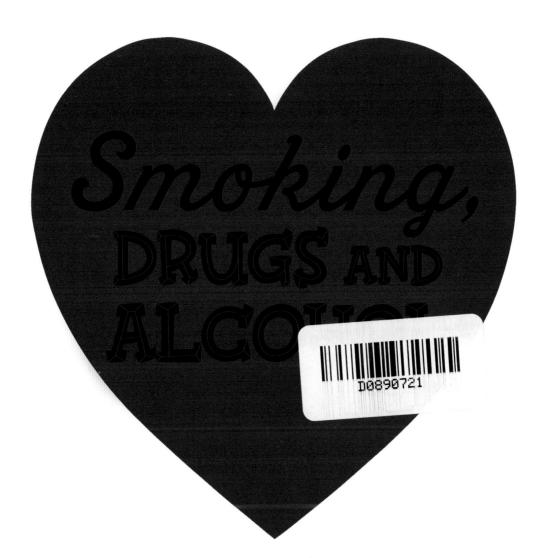

Smoking, DRUGS AND ALCOHOL

Anna Claybourne

W
FRANKLIN WATTS
LONDON•SYDNEY

Franklin Watts
Published in paperback in Great Britain in 2018 by The Watts Publishing Group

Credits
Series editor: Sarah Peutrill
Editor: Sarah Ridley
Art director: Peter Scoulding
Series design and illustrations: Dan Bramall
Cover design: Cathryn Gilbert

Additional pictures by Shutterstock.com

Every attempt has been made to clear copyright. Should there be any inadvertent
omission please apply to the publisher for rectification.

ISBN 978 1 4451 4976 9

Printed in China

MIX
Paper from
responsible sources
FSC® C104740
www.fsc.org

Franklin Watts
An imprint of
Hachette Children's Group
Part of The Watts Publishing Group
Carmelite House
50 Victoria Embankment
London EC4Y 0DZ
An Hachette UK Company
www.hachette.co.uk

www.franklinwatts.co.uk

**Medical, illegal
and recreational
drugs (including alcohol)
are discussed in this
book. The author and
publishers in no way
condone the use or
misuse of drugs
of any sort.**

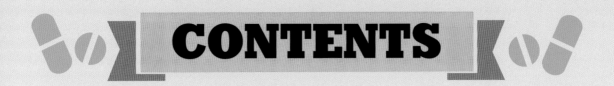

CONTENTS

What are drugs?

'Drugs' is a word that can make you feel scared. You may have heard phrases like 'drugs ruin lives' or 'the war on drugs'. It's true that some drugs are dangerous, but that's not the whole story.

> So what is a drug?

> A drug is a chemical that has an effect on your body and how it works.

There are many, many different types of drugs, used by people in different ways for different reasons. Here are some of them.

MEDICAL DRUGS

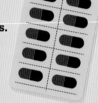

When you take a medicine, you are taking a drug that can help fix a particular problem with your body. Here are two everyday examples.

An asthma inhaler releases a drug that acts on the lungs of someone with asthma, helping their lungs work better.

Painkilling medicines such as paracetamol block pain, which helps to get rid of a headache, for instance.

RECREATIONAL DRUGS

Recreation means enjoyment, and a recreational drug is one that you take because you enjoy it.

Caffeine, found in coffee and tea, is one example. It can help you feel more awake and alert, and many people enjoy its effects every day, as well as enjoying the taste of coffee and tea.

ILLEGAL DRUGS

Most drugs can be harmful if you have too much of them. Some recreational drugs can be especially dangerous, and are banned in most countries.

Well-known illegal recreational drugs include cannabis, heroin and cocaine.

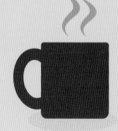
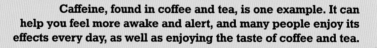
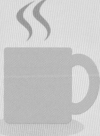
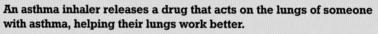
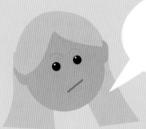
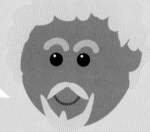
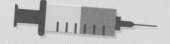

Drug addiction

Drug addiction means wanting, or needing, to keep taking a a drug, and finding it very hard to stop.

Nicotine, found in tobacco, is very addictive – it's easy for people's bodies to start feeling they can't do without it. That's why it can be very hard to kick the smoking habit.

Some medical drugs are addictive too. Doctors are careful to control how much of these drugs their patients take.

Being addicted to a drug can make you very ill and unhappy. It can affect your behaviour, and damage your health (depending on the drug). Sometimes, addiction makes people spend all their money on illegal drugs, leaving them homeless. This is partly why it's important to learn about drugs and how to stay healthy around them.

Taking drugs

To work, drugs have to get into your body.
This can happen in several ways.

In a drink
For instance, coffee contains caffeine – and wine contains alcohol.

In something solid you swallow
For example, a painkilling pill contains paracetamol (or another drug) – and a piece of chocolate contains small amounts of theobromine.

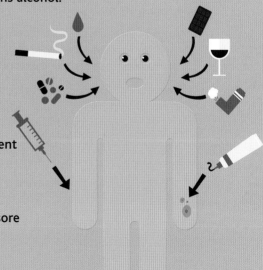

In an injection
For instance, anaesthetics contain drugs that put a patient to sleep – and some recreational drugs are injected.

Through your skin or body surface
For example, some eye drops contain a drug to soothe sore eyes – and some skin creams contain antihistamine to combat an allergic reaction.

Inhaling
Inhalers contain asthma-relief drugs – and cigarette smoke contains nicotine.

Medical drugs

There are thousands and thousands of medical drugs, used to treat all kinds of illnesses and conditions. But while they often save lives, we have to be careful with them too. They can be addictive, or cause other problems.

Where does medicine come from?

Long ago, people knew that some plants could be used as medicines. For example, people in Australia have used tea tree oil to treat cuts and wounds since ancient times. Now, we know it contains powerful germ-killing chemicals, and it is used around the world for its antiseptic and healing powers.

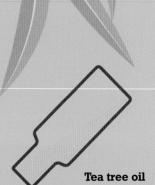

Tea tree plant

Over time, healers, doctors and chemists have studied many traditional plant medicines, and discovered which chemicals they contain, and how they work. Researchers are still investigating plant chemicals to see if they can be used to make new medical drugs.

Tea tree oil

Pestle and mortar for grinding dried plant parts into medicines

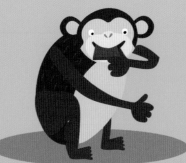

Even chimpanzees use plant medicines. They have learnt to eat certain plant leaves to cure infections, and the bark of the natal fig tree to cure diarrhoea!

Once a new drug has been discovered and tested, chemists work out how to replicate it in a laboratory so that large amounts of the drug can be made. Research chemists also experiment by mixing chemicals to try to discover new drugs that can help different medical conditions.

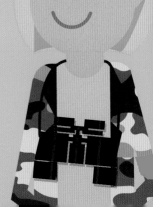

Take care!

Medical drugs can be very powerful. Although they are meant to help us, they can also cause health problems, so they have to be carefully controlled.

Drug safety

In most countries, medicines have to be carefully safety tested before they can be used. There are strict instructions about how much of the drug to take. Taking too much – called an overdose – can be dangerous or deadly.

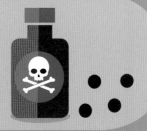

Side effects

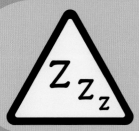

Medical drugs can also be harmful because of their side effects. Any drug can have side effects: it may help to heal your body but also affect you in other less helpful ways. For instance, some antihistamine drugs help with hay fever but also make you feel sleepy or dizzy. That could be bad news if you need to take an exam, or play an important sports match.

Addiction

Some medical drugs can be addictive. They include some painkillers, like codeine and diamorphine, and sedatives (drugs that calm you down) like valium. If you get addicted, you can feel very ill if you try to stop taking the drug.

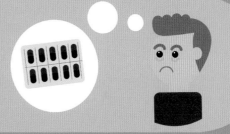

Prescriptions

You can buy some medicines 'over the counter' in a pharmacy or shop. Others you can only get 'on prescription', meaning a doctor or other health professional has to decide that it is what you need, and writes a note saying you can have it. This is to try to control the use of medicines and to stop people from being able to buy too much of an addictive medicine.

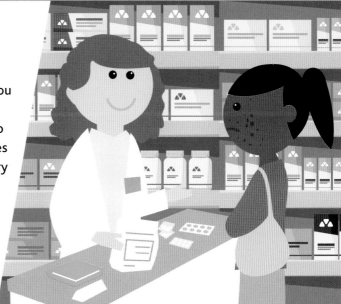

Recreational drugs

Recreational drugs are drugs that are taken for pleasure – and there's nothing new about that. In fact, it's been going on for thousands of years. It's very normal behaviour for adult humans, and almost everyone does it in one way or another.

Brain drugs

Most recreational drugs are 'psychoactive'. That means they affect not just your body, but also your brain by changing how you feel.

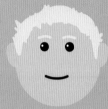

For example, nicotine, the drug in cigarette tobacco, makes people feel calmer and less stressed.

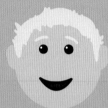

A small amount of alcohol can make people feel relaxed, happy and giggly.

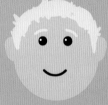

Caffeine in coffee and tea makes people feel more awake and alert, and ready to face the day.

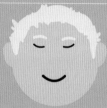

The highly addictive illegal recreational drug, heroin, dulls pain and makes people feel warm and sleepy.

Drug dreams

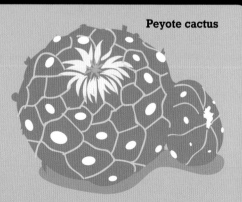

Peyote cactus

Peyote is a drug that comes from a type of cactus. People in Mexico have used it for thousands of years to put them into a thoughtful, dreamy state that sometimes gives them colourful visions too.

Many people around the world have used drugs like peyote as part of religious rituals. This could be because the strange effects some drugs have on the mind can make things seem supernatural or magical.

Everyday drugs and health

Many everyday recreational drugs are legal, but they can still be bad for your health.
Some are always harmful. Other recreational drugs can be safe if you don't have too much.

CIGARETTES

A hundred years ago, cigarettes were sold as a health product that was meant to be good for your throat. But eventually, doctors and scientists realised that smokers were more likely to get serious diseases.

Smoking hasn't yet been banned, but governments try hard to reduce the number of smokers, by helping them give up, as it's so bad for their health.

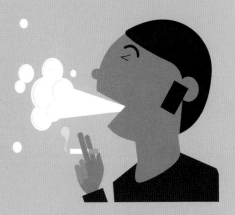

ALCOHOL

Many people drink alcohol without it causing too much damage, although it can make certain diseases, such as cancer, more likely. As long as you are an adult, and only drink small amounts of alcohol, it is safer than many other drugs.

However, alcohol can be very addictive, and this affects some people more than others.

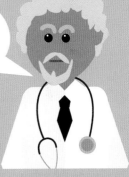

Drinking too much alcohol can damage the liver, an important body organ.

CAFFEINE

Caffeine is a hugely popular drug that's enjoyed around the world. For most people, a few cups of tea or coffee a day are not a problem.

But some people do get addicted to caffeine, and too much can make them tense, or make it hard to sleep. It can also be bad for people who have stomach or anxiety problems.

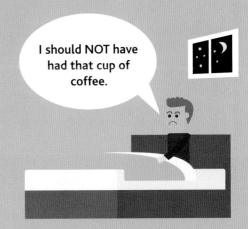

I should NOT have had that cup of coffee.

Alcohol

Humans first made alcoholic drinks, by fermenting fruit and grains, as long as 9,000 years ago. It's one of the world's favourite drugs, especially on social occasions. Like other drugs, though, alcohol comes with a health warning.

How it works

Alcohol is a liquid, so it's usually found in drinks.

Step 1:
When a person drinks alcohol, it goes down into their stomach and intestines.

Step 2:
Some alcohol is soaked up through the stomach. Some is soaked up by the intestines.

Step 3:
From there, alcohol goes into the blood. The blood carries it around the body.

Step 4:
In the brain, the alcohol affects brain cells. It slows down the way they send signals, so it gets harder for the brain to think, understand things and control the body.

What happens?

A small amount of alcohol can just make people feel happy and relaxed. Drinking more and more, though, makes people 'drunk', and this can have more serious effects.

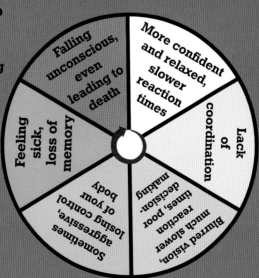

More confident and relaxed, slower reaction times

Lack of coordination

Blurred vision, much slower reaction times, poor decision-making

Sometimes aggressive, losing control of your body

Feeling sick, loss of memory

Falling unconscious, even leading to death

Look at the diagram (left) to find out what happens to someone's body as they drink more and more alcohol. Start with the effect of one drink, printed on white. How quickly someone is affected by alcohol depends on many factors, including what they've eaten that day and whether they drink regularly.

Alcohol and age

When you're a teenager, your brain is still growing and forming, so alcohol can have an even more harmful effect on you than it would on an adult.

That's why, in many countries, there are age limits on when you can legally buy and drink alcohol. For instance, in the UK and Australia you have to be 18 to buy alcohol.

Alcohol emergency

Drinking a lot in one go is called binge drinking, and it can be very dangerous. If someone has too much alcohol, they may become very ill or even unconscious. If you see these signs (below), it's time to get help or call an ambulance:

- Unable to stand up
- Unable to speak clearly
- Breathing oddly
- Looking pale or feeling icy cold
- Falling unconscious

Alcoholism

An alcoholic is addicted to alcohol, which means it is very hard for them to stop drinking it. As well as the effects of being drunk, living with alcoholism over a long period of time can cause heart and liver damage, stomach and throat diseases, weak bones and memory problems.

Alcoholic drinks

There are many different alcoholic drinks, and some contain much more alcohol than others.

Low-alcohol lager
1–2 per cent

Cider
2–8 per cent

Lager
4–6 per cent

Alcopops
4–16 per cent

Wine
10–16 per cent

Sherry
15–20 per cent

Liqueurs
20–50 per cent

Vodka
35–50 per cent

Gin
40–50 per cent

Brandy
40–60 per cent

Whisky
40–70 per cent

Alcohol is sometimes measured in units.

Glass of wine = about 2–3 units

Pint or 500 ml beer = about 2 units

Drinking any amount of alcohol is not good for your body, but people can keep the damage to a minimum by not drinking too much. Experts recommend people should drink no more than two units a day, or 14 units a week. They also advise that two or three days a week should be alcohol free – and alcohol-free weeks are a good idea too.

Smoking

Smoking means inhaling the smoke of tobacco leaves through a lit cigarette, cigar or pipe. It's a popular recreational drug, but it is becoming less common.

Nicotine

The drug involved in smoking is called nicotine, and it is found in the leaves of the tobacco plant.

From tobacco plant to cigarette

Tobacco plant

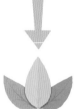

The leaves are dried.

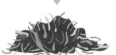

They are shredded into small pieces.

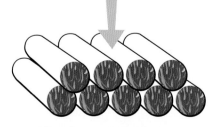

The pieces are rolled up in paper to make cigarettes.

To smoke a cigarette, the smoker sets light to one end, and sucks the smoke from the burning leaves through the other end.

The heart pumps the blood around the body. When it reaches the brain, the nicotine gives the smoker a calm, relaxed feeling.

Smoking sucks the smoke into the lungs, where the nicotine in it passes straight into the blood.

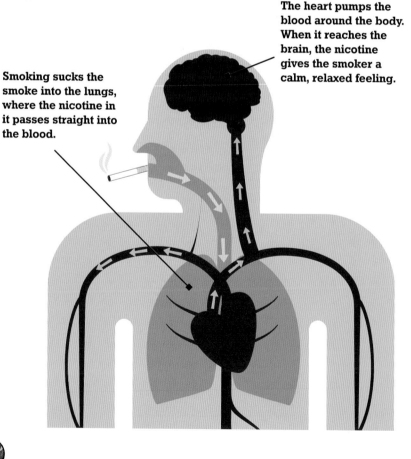

Smoke damage

The smoke from the tobacco leaves contains many other chemicals, as well as nicotine. They harm the lungs, and also make it harder to take in the oxygen the body needs.

Nicotine itself is very addictive. That means people get hooked on smoking and find it hard to stop. People who smoke for years damage their body and are more likely to develop several illnesses. They include: asthma, emphysema, lung cancer and other cancers (such as throat and stomach cancer), heart disease and stroke.

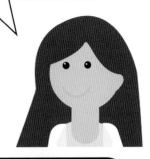

Smoking can also make people's breath and clothes smelly, and harm their teeth, gums and skin.

Quit smoking!

Giving up smoking can be difficult, but it's getting easier. There are now nicotine patches, chewing gum and tablets that give people nicotine without the smoke. Using these, smokers can gradually cut down and stop. The good news is that when people give up, their health improves. Their lungs recover and after a while, they can go back to normal.

As the dangers of smoking become better known, fewer people are starting in the first place. In many parts of the world, the number of smokers is falling, year by year.

E-cigarettes and vaping

An e-cigarette is an electronic cigarette containing a liquid, which it makes into a vapour that the user inhales, or 'vapes'. The vapour usually contains nicotine, but may just contain flavourings, such as vanilla or cherry. Some e-cigarettes look like cigarettes, while others look like pens.

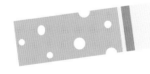

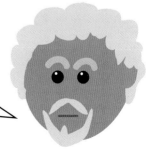

It isn't clear yet how safe vaping is – so it is not a good idea to try it if you don't smoke. However, for people who are already smokers, it does seem to be safer than smoking tobacco and helps some people quit smoking.

Legal highs

Legal highs are a type of recreational drug that is not officially illegal. They are designed to have similar effects to illegal drugs such as cocaine or ecstasy (see pages 18–19). Just because they are described as 'legal' does not make them safe to use.

Why 'high'?

A 'high' describes the effects of taking a recreational drug – whether that means feeling excited, happy or sleepy, or seeing hallucinations. It's normally used to talk about the effects of illegal drugs on the human body. A legal high is a drug that's similar to an illegal drug, but has not yet been banned.

What they look like

Legal highs can be sold in several forms, in shops or online.

A liquid designed to be sniffed (such as poppers)

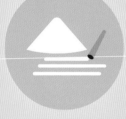

Powders for inhaling or snorting

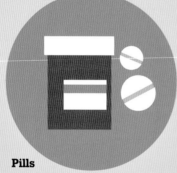

Pills

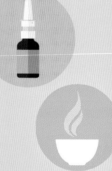

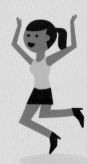

Leaves for making into a kind of tea

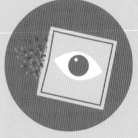

Smoking mixtures to smoke in a similar way to tobacco

Effects

Different legal highs have different effects. Typically, they try to mimic illegal drugs. This could result in different feelings.

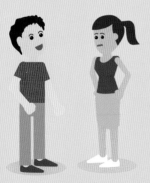

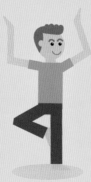

- Feeling wide awake, chatty, witty and confident – similar to the effects of cocaine.

- Feeling relaxed, good-natured and humorous – similar to the effects of cannabis (or marijuana).

- Feeling overjoyed, loving, caring and excited – similar to the effects of ecstasy.

Are they safe?

Unfortunately, legal does not mean safe. There have been many reports of legal highs causing health problems and even deaths. This is for several reasons.

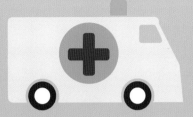

1. They are often new and untested. At first, no one knows what the side effects will be and these can turn out to be serious, such as heart failure, overheating or falling into a coma.

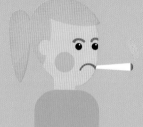

2. Drugs affect different people in different ways. So one person could use a legal high and feel OK, while another might become very ill or die.

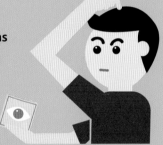

3. Unlike food and medicines, the sale of legal highs is not controlled by regulations. That means the drug could be mixed with something else, or even be something completely different from what the label says.

Legal or not?

Legal highs are substances that are not illegal in themselves. But it IS often illegal to sell them as a drug or as a food, as this would mean they would have to pass safety tests. So they are often sold with warnings on them, telling you not to swallow or smoke them. (Even though that is actually what people do.)

New legal highs are always being created in laboratories, and some become widely used. Often, they turn out to be harmful, and then governments set about banning them. The smoking mixture, Spice, for example, and the drug mephedrone (also called M-cat), were once legal highs. Now they are illegal in many countries.

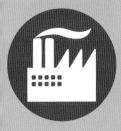
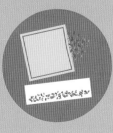
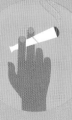
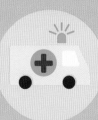
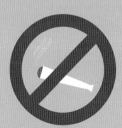

Sniffing

Another type of 'legal high' involves sniffing or inhaling (or 'huffing') solvents, a type of substance found in common products, such as glue or paint.

Everyday chemicals

These substances are sold for other reasons, so they are easy to buy in shops or even find at home. For example:

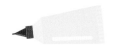

Strong glue is sold for woodworking.

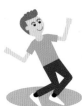

Lighter fuel is sold for filling cigarette lighters and blowtorches.

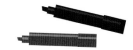

There are strong solvent chemicals in some varnishes, marker pens and nail polish.

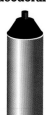

Aerosols might be used in hairsprays, spray paint or deodorant.

What happens?

People sometimes sniff or inhale these substances directly. Alternatively they may soak a cloth in the substance and put it over their face, or put the substance inside a plastic bag and sniff from that.

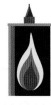

The effects are often described as a short 'rush' of feeling excited, happy, confused, 'drunk', dizzy or dreamy.

Sometimes, people become angry, aggressive or depressed, or just feel sick.

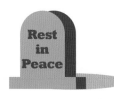

Sniffing can make some people faint or develop very bad headaches.

In rare cases it has caused sudden deaths by stopping the heart.

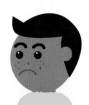
Rest in Peace

There is also a risk of suffocation from people falling unconscious with the bag or cloth over their face.

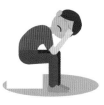

Sniffers can get a rash around their nose and mouth.

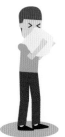

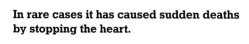

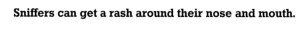

Unknown dangers

As with other legal highs, sniffing can be dangerous because people don't always know how they will react to the substance. One person might not feel very much at all, while another might have a bad reaction, or react differently because they already have a heart problem or asthma, for instance.

It's hard to control these products, as people need them for their main purpose, such as glueing wood. But in many countries there are laws to prevent people under a certain age buying them.

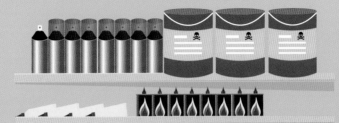

PROOF OF AGE NEEDED TO BUY THESE PRODUCTS

Nitrous oxide

Nitrous oxide, also called laughing gas or 'hippy crack', is a gas that can be used as a medical drug, to help relieve pain in hospital or at the dentist. It's also used in whipped cream dispensers.

Nitrous oxide has been used as a recreational drug for over two hundred years. Today people inhale it from small metal canisters or pre-filled party balloons. Inhaling it can make people feel very happy and giggly. However, it can also be dangerous, as too much of the gas blocks oxygen from getting into the lungs, meaning users can suffocate. Also, people cannot always be sure what gas they are inhaling, so they might inhale something much more dangerous.

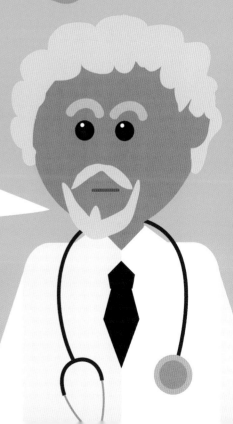

Nitrous oxide is also dangerous when combined with drinking alcohol.

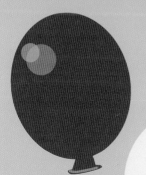

Illegal drugs

In most countries, there's a long list of drugs that are completely illegal. Some can be used as medicines but are banned as recreational drugs. Many are very addictive and have led to countless deaths.

These are some of the best-known illegal drugs.

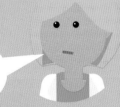

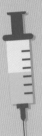

Heroin (also known as smack, skag, gear)

Form: white or brown powder that's usually smoked or turned into a liquid and injected

Effects: feeling numb, warm, relaxed and sleepy

Risks: coma, inhaling vomit, breathing problems

Cocaine (also known as coke, charlie, snow, crack)

Form: white powder or crystals (crack) that can be inhaled, smoked or injected

Effects: feeling energetic, chatty and confident, talking very fast

Risks: overheating, heart problems, nose damage

Cannabis (also known as marijuana, weed, dope, pot, hash, skunk, grass)

Form: resin or leaves that can be smoked in a pipe or a cigarette, or eaten

Effects: feeling relaxed, happy, dreamy, giggly but also paranoid and anxious

Risks: scary hallucinations, panic, mental illness, memory loss

Ecstasy (also known as XTC, E, MDMA)

Form: pills or powder that can be snorted or smoked

Effects: feeling energetic, happy, affectionate or anxious

Risks: overheating, heart problems, mental illness

Speed (also known as whizz, amphetamine)

Form: powder or putty that can be swallowed, snorted or injected

Effects: feeling energetic, excited or jumpy

Risks: sleeplessness, heart problems, mental illness

LSD (also known as acid)

Form: squares of paper ('tabs'), or a liquid that can be swallowed

Effects: hallucinations, confusion, intense feelings

Risks: panic attacks, flashbacks, mental illness

Ketamine (also known as K, special K)

Form: powder or tablets that can be snorted or swallowed

Effects: numbness, floating feeling, hallucinations

Risks: injuries (because of feeling no pain), paralysis, incontinence

Drug dealers

Illegal drugs can't be sold in shops. Instead they are bought from criminal drug dealers, and it can be dangerous to get involved with these people.

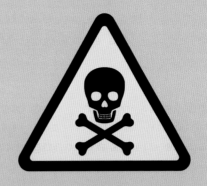

Drug dangers

Illegal drugs cause a lot of health problems. Besides the risks of each drug, there are other dangers:

Addiction

Many illegal drugs, especially heroin, are addictive. They can also be expensive, so addicts spend huge amounts of money on them. Sometimes dealers 'push' drugs, or give them away free, to get users addicted. Then they make money from the users for years by keeping them supplied.

Impurities

Illegal drugs are not regulated or safety checked. It is hard to tell whether they have been mixed with other chemicals that are even more dangerous to put into your body.

Overdoses

It's hard for users to know the strength of an illegal drug, so it can be easy to accidentally take too much, known as an overdose.

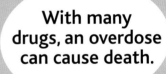

With many drugs, an overdose can cause death.

Injecting

Injecting drugs carries extra health risks. Sharing needles can spread dangerous diseases such as AIDS and hepatitis. It can also damage blood vessels and skin.

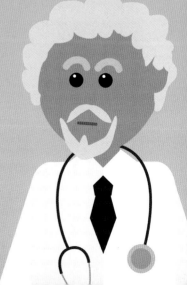

Problems with drugs

Drugs are obviously a big part of our lives – as medicines, and in normal ways like drinking coffee. But when things go wrong, drugs can cause misery and chaos. That's why parents, schools and governments worry about them so much.

The impact of drugs

Drugs are most likely to have a bad effect when people become addicted to them, or experiment and take risks with recreational drugs.

DRUG DEATHS

Sadly, people do die from drug use. This can be due to:

- Accidental drug overdoses
- Taking impure drugs that contain other dangerous substances
- Allergic reactions
- Risky behaviour after drug taking, such as jumping in a lake.

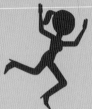

ADDICTION IMPACTS

Someone who is seriously addicted to a drug will do anything to get more of it. The drug can also affect their behaviour.

- Addicts may spend all their money on drugs, and have none left for food or housing.
- Addicts may struggle with school work, or lose their job, because they cannot function well.
- Addicts may commit crimes such as robbery to get money for drugs.

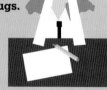

FAMILIES AND RELATIONSHIPS

Drug addicts can behave very selfishly, because the drug matters more to them than anything else. They can be very difficult to live with.

- People can lose touch with their families.
- Relationships can break up.
- Parents who are drug addicts often fail to care for their children properly, which can lead to family breakdown.
- When someone is using drugs, they can say things which upset family, friends and neighbours.

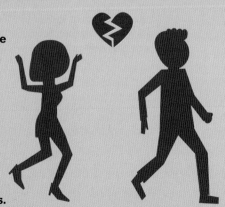

LONG-TERM HEALTH

Many drugs, such as cocaine, cannabis and speed, can have a negative long-term effect on the brain or body, especially if they are used heavily.

- Drug users can develop depression, anxiety or other mental illnesses.
- The drug may damage their memory or learning skills.
- Drugs can also damage the heart, liver, throat and other body parts.

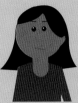

A CRIMINAL RECORD

With illegal drugs, buying, selling or owning them can get users into trouble with the law.

- Being convicted of a crime can make it hard to get a job.
- Spending time in prison can lead to more drug use.

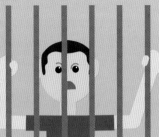

What can you do?

Problems can develop with the use of both illegal drugs, and legal ones such as alcohol or legal highs. But with illegal drugs, people can be more afraid to ask for help because they have broken the law.

However, if you think you or anyone you know might have a drug problem, it's always better to tell someone – maybe a doctor, trusted family friend or parent.
They should be able to help.

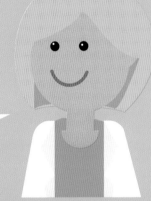

Lots of people have recovered from drug addiction, and live normal, happy lives.

Drug emergency

If you're with friends and someone becomes ill or unconscious after taking drugs, it's important to get help at once. Even if it's an illegal drug, do call an ambulance. It also helps to tell the ambulance staff what the person took, how much of it they took, and show them some of it if possible. This can help doctors give the person the best possible treatment.

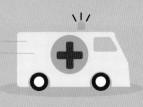

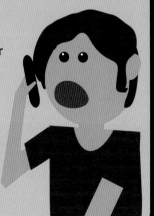

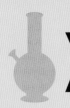

Peer pressure

Your 'peers' are your equals – people you know who are a similar age to you, such as your friends, classmates or siblings.

What is peer pressure?

Peer pressure is pressure from peers to behave in certain ways. This could be about things like what to wear, what music is 'in', or whether to go to a certain party.

Sometimes peer pressure involves teasing, bullying or just telling you what to do.

Sometimes it's more subtle: classmates leaving you out if you're a bit different, or making you feel uncool if you don't have the 'right' clothes.

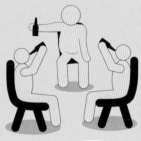

I don't want to get drunk, but they're my friends.

Peer pressure and drugs

Peer pressure can also play a part in teenagers experimenting with cigarettes, alcohol and other drugs. People often try drugs because other people are, and they don't want to be left out. Or their peers may try to persuade them to do it – and laugh at them if they don't.

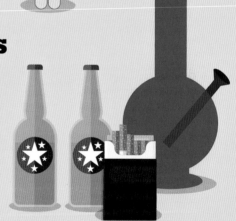

Why does it happen?

Peer pressure actually comes from worry and insecurity. Most people don't like being the odd one out. If they want to try something risky or illegal, they feel better if they can persuade others to do it too.

Resisting peer pressure

There are several ways to resist peer pressure if you don't want to do something.

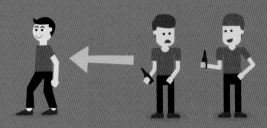

You have the right to say 'no' to drinking, smoking or drug taking. You don't have to give a reason why.

Choose your friends

No one has to hang out with friends who pressure them or make them feel uncomfortable. It's OK to switch to other groups of friends, or just be 'too busy'.

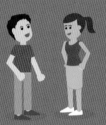

Be proud of what you want

It can be scary to simply say: 'No, I don't want to' or 'I'm not into that'. However, people often find that if they are brave enough to do that, others actually respect it, or even copy them.

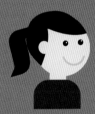

Handy excuses

It does take a lot of confidence to stand up to peer pressure. If you don't feel able to, excuses can work too. Here are a few ideas to try out.

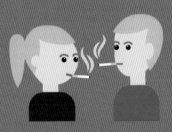

- You have a health condition like asthma or allergies, and drugs aren't safe for you.

- You're dedicated to your sport, dance or music, and drugs could ruin your performance.

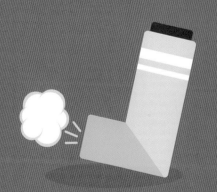

- You don't want to upset your fantastic parents.

- You're scared to upset your strict parents.

- You don't agree with the way the drugs trade exploits people (see pages 24–25).

Where do drugs come from?

Legal drugs, like cigarettes and alcoholic drinks, are made in factories and sold in shops according to strict regulations. But illegal drugs, and some legal highs, are a different story.

When someone buys drugs on the street, from a friend, or over the Internet, that drug may have come on a long journey.

Growing

Drugs like heroin are made from plants grown in other countries, often far away.

Manufacturing

Drugs such as ecstasy and speed are made in illegal factories in various parts of the world.

Workers

People who grow or make drugs are often very poorly paid, and can be mistreated by their employers. If they are making something illegal, it's hard for them to complain or get help.

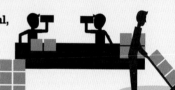

Transport

If it's illegal to bring a drug into a country, it may be smuggled in instead. People may be bullied or pressured into carrying drugs in their luggage or even inside their bodies (see page 25).

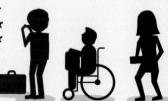

Drugs trade

Drugs are bought and sold as they move around the world from one dealer to the next. With so much money at stake, drug dealers can be violent and dangerous. They may threaten each other and have 'turf wars' over territory.

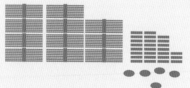

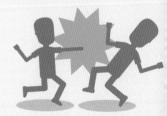

Drug user

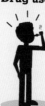

Drugs mules

A drugs mule is someone who illegally carries drugs from one place to another – usually to smuggle them into a country. Sometimes, very poor people become drugs mules for money. Others are forced to become mules by drug dealers.

If someone gets caught smuggling drugs, they face prison or, in some countries, the death penalty.

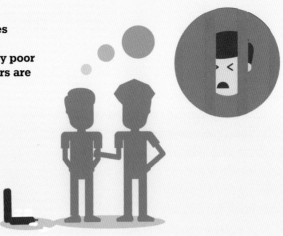

Sometimes drugs mules swallow packets of drugs, such as cocaine, complete the journey, then poo out the packets and collect them.

But the packets can burst in the person's stomach, killing them with an overdose.

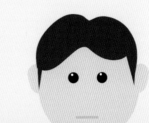

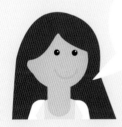

This is one reason you are always asked if you have packed your own bags at aiports. It's very unwise to carry a bag or parcel for anyone.

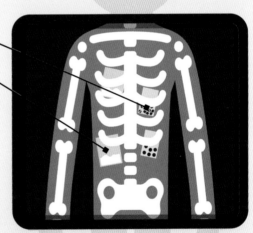

It's not fair!

As you can see, the way illegal drugs reach their destination is the opposite of fair trade. The drugs trade only exists to make money. Illegal drugs are unregulated, so it's hard to make sure the people involved are treated well. And those who deal in drugs are often ruthless criminals – they don't care if people get hurt or die along the way. They just want drug users to get addicted, so that they will keep on buying.

Healthy for life

Drugs of various types are almost certainly going to play a significant part in your life. Most people enjoy tea, coffee, alcohol or chocolate, and reach for a pill if they have a headache or hay fever. If you get very ill, medical drugs might even save your life.

So drugs are not all bad. It's just that some drugs are dangerous, while others can be bad news if they are used in certain ways. So it's useful to know how to keep yourself safe and out of trouble.

Be informed

The information in this book is here to help you understand all the different types of drugs, what they do, and what problems they can cause – so that you can make your own decisions and know what you're talking about.

It's your life and your body, and it's your choice how you look after it and what you put into it.

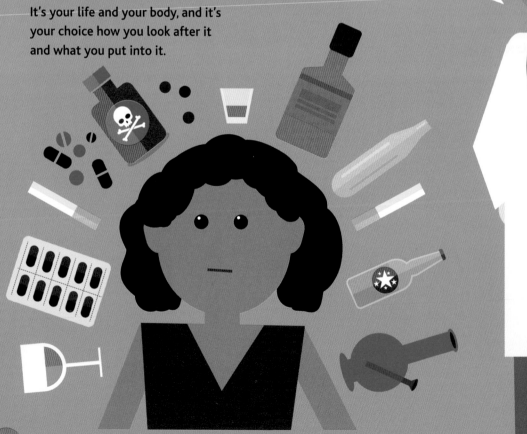

Your choice – not your peers', a drug dealer's, or anyone else's!

Turning to drugs

Most people will have times in their lives when they feel sad, overwhelmed, worried or angry. They might be very sad after the death of a loved one, be suffering from depression or anxiety, their parents might be splitting up, or they may be failing at something that matters to them.

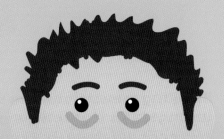

At times like these, some people are more likely to try illegal drugs, or misuse drugs (by drinking too much alcohol, for example). This is partly because drugs often have a numbing, soothing or distracting effect – but obviously, forgetting about your problems for a little while won't solve them.

In addition, as this book shows, getting addicted to drugs or using illegal drugs can make people ill and make their problems far worse. It's better to look for help with unhappy feelings than to use drugs to help mask the real issues.

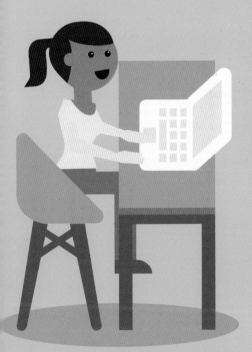

Find out more

It's not possible to fit all there is to know about drugs into a short book like this. If you need to know more about particular types of drugs you might be worried about, or about how to get help for someone, there are lots of useful websites you can use. Some of them are listed at the back of this book (see page 31).

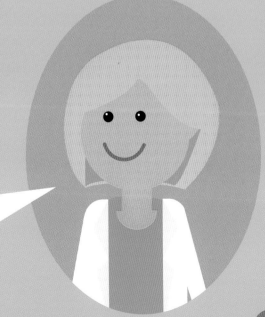

A doctor is a good person to ask when looking for advice!

Types of drugs

Here's a selection of some of the drugs you may have heard of, and what they all do.

Common medical drugs

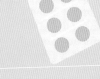

Drug:	Used to treat:
Paracetamol	Pain and fever
Ibuprofen	Pain and inflammation
Aspirin	Pain, inflammation and fever
Codeine	Pain
Diamorphine	Pain
Antihistamines	Hay fever and allergies
Valium	Anxiety
Benzoyl peroxide	Acne
Hydrocortisone	Eczema
Diphenhydramine (Benadryl)	Travel sickness
Corticosteroids	Asthma, eczema, inflammatory diseases
Antibiotics, such as penicillin	Bacterial infections
Insulin	Diabetes
Statins	High cholesterol

Legal recreational drugs (in most countries)

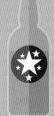
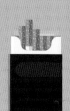

Drug:	Effects:
Alcohol	Happy mood, slow reactions, sleepiness
Nicotine	Calm mood, relaxation, alertness
Caffeine	Wakefulness, alertness, restlessness

Drugs found in foods (in small amounts)

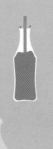
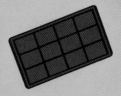

Drug:

Theobromine

Taurine

Opiates (similar to heroin)

Quinine

Dopamine

Caffeine

Found in:

Chocolate

Energy drinks

Poppy seeds

Tonic water

Bananas

Tea and coffee

Illegal recreational drugs (in most countries) and legal highs

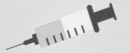

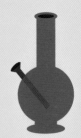

Drug:

Heroin

Cocaine/Crack

Cannabis

Ecstasy/MDMA

Speed/Amphetamine

LSD/Acid

Ketamine

Crystal meth

Mephedrone/M-Cat

PCP/Angel dust

Solvents

Nitrous oxide/Hippy crack

Effects:

Numbness, sleepiness, relaxed mood, dizziness, sickness

Excitement, confidence, chattiness, jitteriness

Happy and giggly mood, relaxation, sleepiness, sickness, anxiety and paranoia

Excitement, energy, friendliness, thirstiness, overheating

Wakefulness, jitteriness, confusion

Hallucinations, wonder, confusion, fear

Numbness, floatiness, hallucinations

Wakefulness, energy, aggression, confusion

Alertness, friendliness, anxiety

Floaty, dreamy feeling, numbness, hallucinations, panic

Dizziness, excitement, headaches, sickness

Happiness, laughing, dizziness, sickness

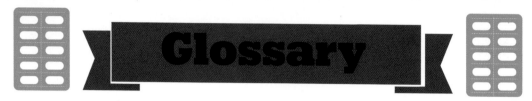

Glossary

addiction Becoming dependent on a drug, so that it is very hard to stop using it.

AIDS (Acquired Immune Deficiency Syndrome) A serious illness caused by a virus that can be spread by sharing needles used for injecting drugs.

allergic reaction A bad reaction to a food, drug or other substance, which can make some people very ill.

asthma A long-term health condition marked by attacks, in which tubes in the lungs become narrower, causing difficulty with breathing. It is usually connected to an allergic reaction or some other trigger.

binge drinking Drinking a lot of alcohol on one day, or in a short space of time.

blood clot A lump of hardened blood.

cancer Disease in which some of the body's cells grow out of control.

coma A state of deep, long-lasting unconsciousness caused by illness or an injury.

drug A substance that has an effect on the way the body works.

drug dealer Someone who sells recreational drugs, usually illegally.

drug pushing Encouraging people to take drugs in order to make them become addicted.

drugs mule Someone who is paid or pressured to carry drugs into a country illegally.

e-cigarette (electronic cigarette) An electronic device used to inhale nicotine or flavoured vapour.

emphysema An illness that damages the lungs and makes it hard to breathe properly.

exploit To use or benefit from someone else in an unfair way.

flashback Suddenly remembering or re-experiencing the effects of being on drugs in the past.

germs Tiny living things that can cause some types of diseases.

hallucination Seeing or experiencing something that is not really there.

hepatitis An illness that damages the liver, an important body organ.

huffing Another name for sniffing or inhaling solvents or gases.

illegal drugs Drugs that are banned by the laws of the country you are in.

incontinence Being unable to control urination (weeing) or defecation (pooing).

inhaler A device that lets you take a medical drug by breathing it in.

legal high A recreational drug that resembles or mimics illegal drugs but is not banned by the laws of a country, although it may well be in due course.

medical drug A drug that is used as a medicine to treat illnesses or health conditions.

mental illness Illness that affects your mind and emotions.

overdose Taking too much of a drug, which can be harmful or fatal.

paralysis Being unable to move all or part of your body.

peer pressure Pressure from your peers – friends, schoolmates or people a similar age to you – to behave in particular ways.

prescription An official instruction from a doctor that allows you to be given a medical drug.

psychoactive drug A drug that changes the way the brain works, and can affect moods, feelings, behaviour or senses.

recreational drug A drug that is taken for enjoyment.

rush A sudden feeling of dizziness, excitement or happiness that can be caused by some drugs.

sedative A drug that calms you down or makes you feel sleepy.

side effects Extra effects that a drug can have as well as its main effect or purpose.

smuggling Bringing a drug or other substance into a country illegally.

snorting Sniffing a drug up the nose in the form of a powder.

solvent A type of substance often found in glue, paint and other products, that can have a drug-like effect when inhaled.

stroke Damage to the brain caused by a blood clot or leak in a blood vessel.

suffocation Being unable to breathe.

turf war A fight between drug dealers over the areas of a town or city where they want to sell drugs.

unconscious Asleep and unaware of anything, and unable to wake up.

unit A measurement of alcohol, equivalent to about half a small glass of wine or half a pint of beer.

vaping Inhaling nicotine vapour or another flavoured vapour using an e-cigarette.

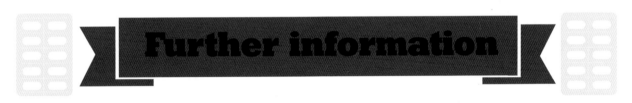

Further information

Books

Buzzed: The Straight Facts About the Most Used and Abused Drugs from Alcohol to Ecstasy
by Cynthia Kuhn, Scott Swartzwelder, Wilkie Wilson, Jeremy Foster and Leigh Heather Wilson, (Norton, 2014)

Keeping Safe Around Alcohol, Drugs and Cigarettes
by Anne Rooney (Franklin Watts, 2014)

Teen FAQ: Alcohol
by Anne Rooney (Franklin Watts, 2010)

The Hidden Story of Alcoholism/Drugs
by Karen Latchana Kenney (Raintree, 2016)

52 Teen Boy/Teen Girl Problems & How to Solve Them
by Alex Hooper-Hudson (Wayland, 2014)

Websites

Frank: Friendly, confidential drugs advice
www.talktofrank.com

TeensHealth: Drugs & Alcohol
kidshealth.org/en/teens/drug-alcohol/

Teen Health: Peer Pressure
www.cyh.com/HealthTopics/HealthTopicDetails.aspx?p=243&id=2184&np=295

The CoolSpot: Alcohol and Peer Pressure
www.thecoolspot.gov

Note to parents and teachers: Every effort has been made by the Publishers to ensure that these websites are suitable for children, that they are of the highest educational value, and that they contain no inappropriate or offensive material. However, because of the nature of the Internet, it is impossible to guarantee that the contents of these sites will not be altered. We strongly advise that Internet access is supervised by a responsible adult.

Index

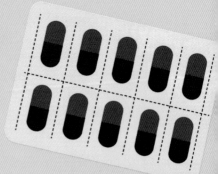